T0171337

The Goodness and Best-Kept *Secrets* of Mediterranean Food

Slow Down the Ageing Process

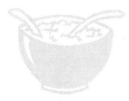

ORTENSIA GRECO-CONTE

BALBOA.
PRESS

A DIVISION OF HAY HOUSE

Balboa Press books may be ordered through booksellers or by contacting:

Balboa Press
A Division of Hay House
1663 Liberty Drive
Bloomington, IN 47403
www.balboapress.com.au
1-(877) 407-4847

ISBN: 978-1-4525-0858-0 (sc)
ISBN: 978-1-4525-0859-7 (e)

Balboa Press rev. date: 02/22/2013

CONTENTS

Four Generations.. xi
Some Healthy and Wise Advice from a Mediterranean Great-Grandma xv

Healthy, fast power food containing natural pharmacologically
protective agents that can defeat some viruses

Spring Salad Wraps...3
Tuna & Ricotta Rolls...4
Fresh Fruit and Prosciutto Wraps 5
Chicken Salad Wraps 6
Whole-Grain Bread Roll Salad 7
Figs with Red Leaf Salad on Pita Bread................................8
Crab and Mushroom Salad..9
Beans and Tomato Salad 10
Nectarine Salad 11
Lentil Salad 12
Lettuce and Tuna Wraps... 13
Mediterranean Salad... 14
Smoked Salmon Rolls 15
Melon and Tofu Mountain Bread 16
Tomato-Olive-Caper Salad.. 17
Smoked Salmon Salad 18
Organic Garden Salad.. 19
Asparagus and Fennel Salad 20
Prawn and Green Salad.. 21
Pasta Salad 22
Steamed Scallop Salad Pasta 23
Ricotta Pasta Salad 24
Feta Cheese Salad.. 25
Chocolate Fruit Wraps... 26
Tropical Fruit Wraps.. 28
Mediterranean Herbed Pasta Salad 29
Sweet Ricotta Wrap 30
Pizza Wraps.. 31
Passionfruit Wraps... 32

Exotic Fruit Salad...33
Sweet Wraps...34
Mozzarella Cheese and Boiled Egg Wraps 35
Sunshine Wraps...36
Mediterranean Antioxidant Couscous................................37
Pumpkin Gnocchi with Ricotta Cheese..............................38
Lasagne Italiana 39
Mediterranean Grilled Salad..41
Mediterranean Minestrone Soup 42
Mixed Tongue Salad..43
Mediterranean Bread Salad...44
Sardine Ripiene (Sardine Sandwich) 45
Marinated Prawns with Italian Herbs.................................46
Fresh Fish with Onions, Capers, and Vinegar
    (Salmon, Trout, Swordfish or Mullet) 47
Light Supper of Apple and Prawn Salad 48
Moussaka..49
Eggs with Ricotta and Vegetable 51
Rice and Potato Soup..52
Mussels Gratinate 53
Fast Fettuccine 54
Quick Tagliatelle with Tuna 55
Meatball Fritters...56
Sweet Pumpkin Chips 57
Rice and Ricotta Fritters...58
Tomato Parmigiana...59
Quick Energy Booster 1: Bruschetta Bread Pizzaiola...........60
Quick Energy Booster 2: Bruschetta Bread with Tomato and Basil........61
Quick Energy Booster 3: Bruschetta Bread with Mushrooms, Tomato,
    and Onions...62
Greek Salad 63
Italian Stuffed Squid...64
Orecchietti with Broccoli and Cauliflower 65
Spaghetti with Aglio E Olio 67
Stuffed Peppers with Antioxidant Couscous.......................68
Tomatoes Stuffed with Rice 69
Octopus, Potato, and Onion Stew 70
Octopus Salad 71
Black Olive Bread..72

How To Preserve Fresh Tomatoes 75
   Date and Zucchini Loaf 76
   Pumpkin Soup with Buttered Bread 77
   Mediterranean Grilled Salad... 78
   Spaghetti Napoletana 79
   Spaghetti with Black Sauce of Cuttlefish and Peas 80
   Spaghetti with Fried Zucchini... 82
   Pasta Al Forno (Baked In Oven) 83
   Tagliatelle Alla Siciliana... 84
   Spaghettini with Eggplant and Tomato Sauce 85
   Sicilian Potato Cakes 86
   Macaroni Siracusa 87
   Pasta Capriccosa.. 88
   Mediterranean Risotto... 89
   Mediterranean Eggs.. 90
   Spaghetti with Meatball Sauce 91
   Tagliatelle Alla Siciliana... 92
   Spaghetti with Prawns 93
   Mediterranean Bread Salad.. 94
   Mediterranean Frittata 95
   Cannelloni with Ricotta and Spinach 96
   Tagliatelle Primavera 99
   Salmon Potato Cakes.. 100
   Fettuccine Carbonara.. 101
   Conchiglioni with Spinach and Ricotta 102
   Healthy Vegetables with Couscous.. 103
   Caponata Siciliana.. 104
   Prawn Salad 106
   Pepperonata with Potatoes 107
   Tofu Pizzaiola.. 108
   Vegetable Lasagne 110
   Mortadella and Onion Pizza Wheels.. 112
   Spinach Ricotta Pizza Wheel 114
   Yummy Italian Arancine 116
   Fusilli Pasta with Tuna and Tomato 118
   Fresh Tuna Marinade 119

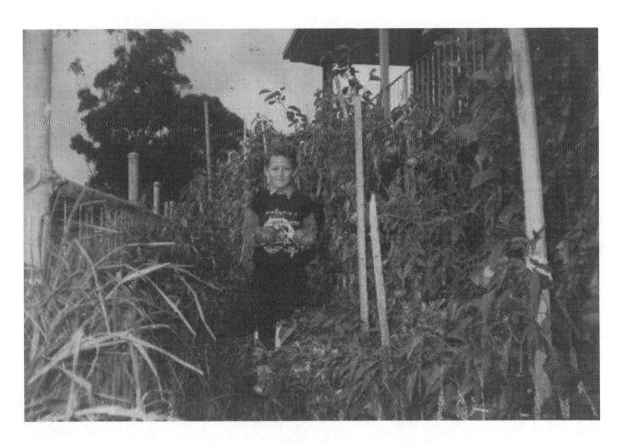

My son Andrew in our vegetable garden.

FOUR GENERATIONS

Dear friends,

I would like to share with you some best-kept secrets and traditional recipes from the Mediterranean people, famous for their longevity and colourful and healthy cuisine. Our grandmothers have always known that Mother Nature stores what our body needs. Evidence shows that *fresh food* is our *best medicine.* For generations, the Mediterraneans have been filling their tables each day with healthy, essential food full of anti-ageing antioxidants such as homemade bread, pasta, fresh organic vegetables picked from the garden, fresh Mediterranean herbs and spices, tomatoes, onions, garlic, basil, extra virgin olive oil, cheese (fresh and *stagionato*), fresh milk and dairy foods, polenta, rice, parsley, mixed salad, capsicum, lemon, eggplant, green and black olives, lentils and all types of legumes, spinach, cereals, nuts, fresh and dry beans, peas, corn, mixed fresh and dry fruit, and all types of fish and seafood, and only once or twice a week eggs, low-fat poultry, and some red meat. Only occasionally do they have take-away food.

Every dish is cooked with the finest extra virgin olive oil. Olive oil lowered blood pressure in a study of twenty thousand people by Harvard and University of Athens researchers. Those with healthy blood pressure averaged three ounces of olive oil a day; blood pressure protection starts with just one ounce a day, experts say. A Harvard study of 732 women showed that atherosclerosis-causing blood chemicals were lowest in those on a Mediterranean diet and highest in those on Western diet. High-antioxidant fruits and vegetables and omega-3-rich fish are heart protective, while trans fats in Western-style fast food irritate blood. So it is very important to eat a traditional Mediterranean diet; all this powerful food provides fuel and energy for our bodies in the form of carbohydrates, fibre, protein, vitamins, and minerals, which are rich sources of antioxidants and anti-ageing.

In some smaller towns, older people live longer and healthier just by the type of foods they eat, as the fruit and vegetables are fresh from their garden, grown without chemicals or pesticides. They prefer to consume fresh food, not much pre-packaged food. Fishing is a popular hobby, so they have fish and all types of seafood daily with their pasta and fresh mixed salad.

The Mediterranean secret to longevity is eating very fresh *organic* food, raw or cooked, and all types of cereals and very fresh fruit and veggies, Older generations of Mediterraneans do not consume much processed foods or packaged foods with nasty additives. Most of their food has no artificial colours, no preservatives or synthetic antioxidants. They prefer homemade food from nature and all things that come from the earth in the season. For example, if they pick some fresh tomatoes, carrots, or broccoli from their own garden today, they will consume it the same day; this is alive, young, active, powerful, fresh antioxidants and beta-carotene, for the rejuvenation of every cell in our bodies. Organic fruits and vegetables eaten soon after picking are higher in compounds that decrease the risk of cancer and heart disease. This best-kept secret can slow down the ageing process. If we keep food for three days in the fridge, it is still good, but the benefit is not the same. This goes for many types of food. A team of researchers at the USDA has developed a scale to assess the antioxidant content of various plant foods that Mediterraneans use in their diet. It's called the ORAC scale, for oxygen radical absorbance capacity. Basically, the ORAC score reflects a food's ability to neutralize cell-damaging free radicals. The higher the score, the better the food helps prevent cancer and helps in staying young:

Plant Food	ORAC Score
Prunes	5,770
Raisins	2,830
Blueberries	2,400
Blackberries	2,036
Kale	1,770
Tomatoes	1,680
Strawberries	1,540
Spinach	1,260

Raspberries	1,220
Brussels sprouts	980
Plums	949
Alfalfa sprouts	930
Broccoli florets	890
Beetroots	840
Oranges	750
Red grapes	739
Red peppers	710
Cherries	670
Onions and Garlic	450
Corn	400

Good nutrition in fresh food is the key to looking young and slowing down the ageing process. In the old days, there was no electricity, no fridge, and no freezer. People survived by consuming fresh, organic, healthy raw food daily or cooking fresh food daily. If they had fresh eggs, they were from free-range chickens, not animals kept in cages. Mediterranean people also drink plenty of fresh water to keep the body hydrated and help the kidneys flush out all the impurities that are collected in the blood. This is essential for Mediterraneans. Research found that drinking plenty of fresh water increased the metabolic rate by 30 percent, and the effect persisted for ninety minutes. One-third of the boost came from the body's effort to warm the water, but the rest is due to the work the body must exert to absorb it. When drinking water, no calories are ingested, but calories are used, so increasing water consumption (instead of soft drinks) to eight glasses per day may help you lose about eight pounds in a year.

In some Mediterranean towns, not everyone has a television or a car, so people don't sit much. They walk or ride a bike almost everywhere. They keep themselves very active, but on summer afternoons, they love to have a thirty-minute nap (siesta). They are surrounded with a lot of green plants and fresh air to breathe. They prefer to live away from pollution. Of course today, we love our fridge, our television, and our car, but this is the secret of the Mediterranean longevity and well-being—fresh, organic, living food and being active. I hope you all enjoy this treasure trove of best-kept secret information and share the recipes in this book with your family and friends. Remember to use this super anti-ageing food wisely. Consult your doctor if you have dietary problems or food allergies.

My dear family and friends, I always hear people say that I look very young for my age, and they think I must have a good life. But it's not like that. I had a very sad childhood. I learned the secret to staying happy and young. I make my life meaningful and enjoyable with positive thinking and by letting the child in me live and have fun, and following our grandmother's Mediterranean diet. Most of our body cells are constantly replaced, renewed and repaired so i learned to repair myself physically, mentally, spiritually and emotionally.

My wish for all of you is to live longer stronger and stay younger, enjoy life, and smile. Life is beautiful.

SOME HEALTHY AND WISE ADVICE FROM A MEDITERRANEAN GREAT-GRANDMA

- Have regular checkups with the doctor, and check to see if you are allergic to any type of food.

- Eat all types of beans, hearty grains, plenty of dark-green, leafy, and colourful seasonal fruit and veggies.

- Eat bread, cereal, rice, pasta, fish, and protein.

- Drink plenty of water to keep yourself hydrated and flush out impurities. Heavenly Father created water to quench our thirst. Water falls from the sky when it rains, not soft drinks! Tell this to your children, and only consume soft drinks occasionally.

- Chew your food at least twenty times before you swallow it.

- Reduce saturated fats such as deep-fried food or cream cakes, and reduce pre-packaged, processed food.

- If you can, avoid these harmful additives. (Numbers to the left are codes assigned to chemical food additives by the European Food Safety Authority.)

    All Artificial Colours

    Preservatives
    200-203 Sorbates
    210-218 Benzoates
    220-228 Sulphites
    280-283 Propionates
    249-252 Nitrates

> Synthetic Antioxidants
> 310-321 Gallates
> 329-321 Tbhq, Bha, Bht
>
> Flavour Enhancers (All 600 Numbers)
> 620-625 Glutamates, including MSG 621
> 627-635 Nucleotides (Sodium Guanylate 627), (Sodium Inosinate 631), (Ribonucleotides 635)
> 636-637 Maltol, Ethyl, L-Leucine
> Yeast Extract, Hvp, Hpp, Hydrolysed Vegetable, Plant, or Soy Protein.

- Do not overeat. You could be cutting your life short.

- If you have a full stomach at night, wait three to four hours before going to bed.

- Avoid reheating food or cooking too much food in the microwave.

- Do not drink alcohol, as it's bad for your liver and brain.

- Do not smoke, and try to avoid smoking areas.

- Avoid caffeinated drinks and drugs; they may cause liver problems and strokes.

- Do not be alone. Get married, and enjoy the company of family, children, and good friends.

- Try to have a regular routine—wake up each morning at the same time; have breakfast, lunch, and dinner at the same time each day; and go to bed at a particular time each night. (Our body and mind love regularity and gentle discipline).

- Exercise daily, whether it be dancing, walking, swimming, or playing with your pet. Stay active, and it will keep you feeling young and alive.

- If you are religious, go to church as much as possible, pray to God, sing hymns, and read religious books. You will feel good spiritually, physically, and mentally.

- Grow a garden that will reward you with beautiful flowers and healthy herbs, fruits, and vegetables.

- When you have time during the day, relax for fifteen to twenty minutes and concentrate on your breathing. Yoga and meditation are very good.

- Try to keep your body posture straight, and make sure your children do the same.

- Have a massage when you can, and least seven to eight hours of sleep at night. To reduce stress anxiety, watch funny movies. Laughing and smiling also help you to have a positive attitude.

- To contribute positive thoughts, we must keep our house with good energy. Our houses can become sick, just as our bodies can. Our homes can become filled with negative energy, which can affect us mentally and physically without us knowing that they are contributing. For example, anger, argument, negative thoughts, intoxication with alcohol or drugs, depression, sickness, smoking, and dirty and untidy homes yield very negative energy. Because of this, chances are that the house is filled with negative energy. A home needs to feel safe, warm, and inviting, so we all must remove the negative energy and create a more positive atmosphere to help us mentally, physically, and spiritually. If you care and respect your body and your home, you will start feeling better, looking younger, and living longer, and people will love to be near your positive, happy energy.

These are wise ideas to pass to your children and grandchildren.

HEALTHY, FAST POWER FOOD CONTAINING NATURAL PHARMACOLOGICALLY PROTECTIVE AGENTS THAT CAN DEFEAT SOME VIRUSES

SPRING SALAD WRAPS

Servings: 4

Ingredients

4 sheets mountain bread
1 ripe avocado, peeled and sliced
30 g fresh, washed baby spinach leaves
1 cucumber, sliced
2 fresh, washed tomatoes, sliced
50 g kalamata olives
50 g walnuts, finely sliced (if not allergic)
2 fresh, washed spring onions, finely chopped
8 slices swiss cheese (2 slices for each wrap)
4 tbsp. blueberries, (1 tbsp. for each wrap)

Directions

Place the ingredients in the middle of the four wraps, then fold at the ends, roll up, cut in half, and serve.

TUNA & RICOTTA ROLLS

Servings: 4

Ingredients

4 whole-grain bread rolls
4 tsp. fresh blueberries (1 tsp. for each roll)
4 fresh, washed lettuce leaves
¾ cup fresh ricotta cheese
100 g tuna in spring water, drained
2 pickled onions, chopped
1 fresh, washed capsicum, finely chopped
1 stalk fresh, washed celery, finely chopped
1 baby cucumber, finely chopped
Black pepper or chilli for more taste

Directions

Cut the tops off the rolls and hollow out the centre. Place lettuce in each roll, and fill up with the rest of the ingredients. Refrigerate until ready to serve.

FRESH FRUIT AND PROSCIUTTO WRAPS

Servings: 4

Ingredients

4 25-cm (10-inch) wraps
175 g prosciutto, finely sliced
4 tsp. blueberries (1 tsp. for each wrap)
1 large orange, finely sliced
2 cups strawberries, sliced
1 cup fresh, washed, sprouted mung beans

Directions

Place the sprouted mung beans over the wraps, then divide prosciutto and the rest of the fresh fruit. Put all the ingredients in the middle of the wraps, fold at the ends; roll up, cut in half, and serve.

CHICKEN SALAD WRAPS

Servings: 4

Ingredients

4 wraps
4 tsp. mayonnaise
1 avocado, sliced
1 cooked chicken breast fillet, sliced
Cos (romaine) lettuce leaves
1 half cucumber, sliced
1 tomato, sliced
salt and pepper

Directions

Spread wraps with mayo; then layer lettuce, chicken, tomato, cucumber, avocado. Season to taste, fold at the ends; roll up, cut in half, and serve.

WHOLE-GRAIN BREAD ROLL SALAD

Servings: 4

Ingredients

4 whole-grain bread rolls
300 g mozzarella cheese, thinly sliced
1 large beetroot, thinly sliced
1 pinch ginger
2 fresh, washed tomatoes, sliced
1 avocado, sliced
15 fresh, washed basil leaves
4 tsp. extra virgin olive oil (1 tsp. for each roll)
pinch sea salt and hot chilli

Directions

Cut each roll in half. Put all the ingredients in, and top off with the olive oil, salt, and chilli. Cover rolls with plastic wrap and set in a cool place till it is time to serve.

FIGS WITH RED LEAF SALAD ON PITA BREAD

Ingredients

8 fresh or dried figs, sliced
4 slices pita bread
250 g bocconcini cheese, sliced
150 g mixed fresh, washed red lettuce
2 large tomatoes, sliced
4 olives, sliced

Directions

Divide all the ingredients and place in the middle of each pita bread; then fold at the ends, roll up, cut in half, and serve.

(Bocconcini is a small ball of mozzarella cheese, the size of an egg. They are often packaged in water and may be made from buffalo milk.)

CRAB AND MUSHROOM SALAD

Servings: 4

Ingredients

6 fresh mushrooms, chopped
300 g fresh crabmeat
1 clove fresh garlic, chopped
1 fresh spring onion, chopped
1 handful fresh mint
1 avocado, chopped
6 fresh lettuce leaves
1 tbsp. fresh lemon juice
50 g walnuts, chopped
2 tbsp. extra virgin olive oil

Directions

Mix all the ingredients in a large bowl; toss very well and serve.

BEANS AND TOMATO SALAD

Servings: 4

Ingredients

500 g mixed beans, ready-cooked
3 large tomatoes, sliced
2 tbsp. fresh parsley, chopped
2 tbsp. fresh basil, chopped
100 g fresh spinach, chopped
50 g fresh celery, chopped
2 tsp. extra virgin olive oil
2 spring onions, chopped
3 tbsp. balsamic vinegar
sea salt (optional)

Directions

Mix all the ingredients in a large bowl; toss well and serve.

NECTARINE SALAD

Servings: 4

Ingredients

4 fresh nectarines, peeled and segmented
100 g baby rocket (arugula)
1 garlic clove, chopped
250 g fresh cherry tomatoes
1 fresh spring onion
2 fresh carrots, chopped
8 bocconcini cheese, sliced
1 tsp. chia seed
1 tsp. LSA mix (linseed, sunflower kernels, and almonds)
1 pinch cayenne pepper
pinch sea salt (optional)
2 tbsp. extra virgin olive oil

Directions

In a large bowl, mix all the ingredients; toss well and serve.

LENTIL SALAD

Servings: 4

Ingredients

100 g brown lentils (cooked according to package instructions)
3 fresh tomatoes, sliced
1 tbsp. chopped fresh mint
4 baby beetroot, sliced
4 pistachio nuts, chopped
1 fresh spring onion, chopped
50 g fresh, washed mixed salad leaves, chopped
2 tbsp. extra virgin olive oil
juice of 1 fresh lemon
pinch cayenne pepper
pinch chia seed
pinch sea salt

Directions

In a large bowl, mix all the ingredients with the cooked lentils; toss well and serve.

LETTUCE AND TUNA WRAPS

Servings: 4

Ingredients

4 bread wraps
185 g tuna, Italian style
½ head savoy cabbage, shredded
6 fresh spinach leaves
1 fresh carrot, chopped
½ tbsp. chopped ginger
½ tbsp. red chilli
1 mango, sliced
1 handful torn basil leaves
½ tsp. chia seeds
½ tsp. LSA (linseed)

Directions

Place all the ingredients in middle of each wrap; fold the ends, roll up, cut in half, and serve.

MEDITERRANEAN SALAD

Servings: 4

Ingredients

3 tbsp. sun-dried tomatoes
2 spring onions, chopped
4 large fresh lettuce leaves
1 fresh mango, sliced
4 pitted kalamata olives
2 capsicum, red and green, thinly sliced
1 small mozzarella, chopped
1 cucumber, finely chopped
3 tbsp. extra virgin olive oil
3 tbsp. balsamic vinegar
1 tsp. chia seeds
6 fresh mint leaves
pinch sea salt

Directions

Mix all the ingredients in a large bowl; toss well and serve.

SMOKED SALMON ROLLS

Servings: 6

Ingredients

6 fresh rolls
6 small smoked salmon, sliced
250 g Philadelphia brand light cream cheese
150 g fresh, washed baby spinach
2 tsp. traditional basil pesto
2 slices pineapple, finely chopped
juice of 1 lemon, freshly squeezed

Directions

Combine cream cheese, baby spinach, basil pesto, and pineapple. Mix well; stir till smooth. Cut rolls and spread in the combined ingredients. Top with sliced smoked salmon and then squeeze the lemon juice and serve.

MELON AND TOFU MOUNTAIN BREAD

Servings: 4

Ingredients

4 slices mountain bread
½ melon, sliced
2 tomatoes, sliced
4 fresh, washed lettuce leaves
150 g extra-firm tofu, chopped finely
12 fresh, washed basil leaves
1 banana, sliced thin

Directions

Place all the ingredients in middle of each piece of bread. Fold at the end, roll up, cut in half, and serve.

TOMATO-OLIVE-CAPER SALAD

Servings: 4

Ingredients

4 fresh, large tomatoes, chopped
40 g pitted and halved kalamata olives
12 fresh basil leaves
3 tbsp. capers
1 bunch fresh, washed arugula lettuce
1 tsp. chia seeds
1 tsp. LSA mix
1 red chilli
2 tbsp. extra virgin olive oil
2 tbsp. fresh lemon juice
sea salt (optional)

Directions

Combine all the ingredients in a bowl; toss and serve with your favourite bread.

SMOKED SALMON SALAD

Servings: 4

Ingredients

100 g smoked salmon, sliced
16 small rounds bocconcini cheese
1 spring onion, chopped
40 g fresh, washed baby spinach
2 tbsp. extra virgin olive oil
1 red chilli, chopped
1 tsp. chia seed
2 tbsp. fresh lemon juice
sea salt (optional)

Directions

In a large bowl, mix the baby spinach, spring onion, chilli, bocconcini, smoked salmon, chia seed, olive oil, and lemon juice. Mix very well and serve.

ORGANIC GARDEN SALAD

Servings: 4

Ingredients

200 g baby beetroot
150 g cherry tomatoes
1 handful fresh mint leaves
1 handful fresh basil leaves
1 tbsp. fresh celery, chopped
1 fresh spring onion, chopped
1 garlic clove, chopped
1 red capsicum, cut into strips
1 handful fresh spinach
3 tbsp. extra virgin olive oil
juice of 1 fresh lemon
1 fresh red chilli, chopped
sea salt (optional)

Directions

In a large bowl, mix all the fresh, organic ingredients. Then add the extra virgin olive oil and the lemon juice. It is now ready to serve.

ASPARAGUS AND FENNEL SALAD

Servings: 4

Ingredients

2 large, fresh fennel bulbs, thinly sliced
1 bunch fresh asparagus, steamed and chopped
50 g fresh mix salad leaves, chopped
200 g cherry bocconcini cheese
1 red chilli, chopped
1 garlic clove, chopped
1 pinch fresh ginger
50 g unsalted cashew nuts, chopped
1 tsp. chia seed
2 tbsp. extra virgin olive oil
sea salt (optional)

Directions

Mix all ingredients in a large bowl; toss well and serve.

PRAWN AND GREEN SALAD

Servings: 4

Ingredients

200 g steamed prawns, peeled and deveined
1 fresh avocado, sliced
50 g fresh baby spinach
2 tbsp. fresh mint
4 green olives, chopped
1 fresh green chilli, chopped
1 fresh celery stalk, chopped
1 green capsicum, chopped
1 tbsp. chia seed
juice of 1 fresh lemon
2 tbsp. extra virgin olive oil
sea salt (optional)

Directions

In a large bowl, mix all the green ingredients; then add prawns, extra virgin olive oil, lemon juice, and salt. Mix very well and serve.

PASTA SALAD

Servings: 4

Ingredients

125 g farfalle pasta, cooked al dente
2 spring onions
1 garlic clove, crushed
2 anchovy fillets, chopped
1 bunch fresh basil, chopped
200 g baby bocconcini cheese
30 g shaved parmesan cheese
1 red chilli, chopped
2 tbsp. extra virgin olive oil
sea salt (optional)

Directions

In a large bowl, mix pasta and remaining ingredients; toss very well and serve.

STEAMED SCALLOP SALAD PASTA

Servings: 4

Ingredients

400 g steamed scallops
125 g ditali pasta, cooked al dente
2 carrots, chopped
1 garlic clove, crushed
1 fresh spring onion, chopped
2 anchovies, chopped
1 red chilli, chopped
2 fresh tomatoes, sliced
1 tbsp. fresh mint
1 bunch fresh basil, chopped
2 tbsp. extra virgin olive oil
2 tbsp. fresh lemon juice
sea salt (optional)

Directions

In a large bowl, mix pasta, scallops, and remaining ingredients. Toss very well and serve.

RICOTTA PASTA SALAD

Servings: 4

Ingredients

125 g small macaroni pasta, cooked al dente
250 g fresh ricotta cheese
2 tbsp. fresh finely shredded basil
2 fresh roma tomatoes
1 fresh spring onion, chopped
1 fresh garlic clove, chopped
1 red capsicum, chopped
1 tsp. chia seed

Directions

In a large bowl, mix macaroni pasta, ricotta, and remaining ingredients; toss very well and serve.

FETA CHEESE SALAD

Servings: 4

Ingredients

    4 fresh tomatoes, sliced
    200 g feta cheese
    50 g pitted and halved kalamata olives
    2 tbsp. capers, rinsed and drained
    1 bunch fresh basil leaves
    2 small cucumbers, sliced
    50 g fresh baby spinach
    1 fresh spring onion, chopped
    2 tbsp. extra virgin olive oil
    1 red chilli, chopped

Directions

Mix all the ingredients very well in a large bowl; toss and serve.

CHOCOLATE FRUIT WRAPS

Servings: 4

Ingredients

4 plain wraps
2 bananas, sliced
2 tbsp. blueberries
2 tbsp. raspberries
1 mango, sliced thin
4 dried prunes, sliced
1 tsp. chia seed
1 tsp. LSA mix
Icing sugar for dusting

For the hot chocolate:

40 g plain dark chocolate, chopped in small pieces
1 tbsp. butter
150 g golden syrup
1 tbsp. cocoa powder
¼ tsp. vanilla essence
2 tsp. cornflour
3 tbsp. milk

Directions

In a large bowl, mix bananas, sliced blueberry, raspberry, sliced mango, prunes, chia seed, and LSA mix.

To make the chocolate sauce, mix cocoa and cornflour in a bowl. Stir in the milk. In a saucepan, put butter, golden syrup, and the chocolate pieces. Heat gently, stirring well until well blended. Add cocoa mixture and bring to gentle boil, continuing stirring, and simmer for 1 minute. Remove from heat, add vanilla essence, and stir very well. Keep warm. Then divide in four parts the fruits, chia, and LSA mix seed, and put into the middle of each wrap. Put the warm chocolate on top, then fold each end of the wraps. Roll up then cut into the middle. Dust with icing sugar and serve.

TROPICAL FRUIT WRAPS

Servings: 4

Ingredients

4 wraps
1 mango, peeled and sliced
1 passion fruit, sliced
1 papaya, sliced
8 fresh strawberries, sliced
3 fresh kiwi fruit, sliced
2 bananas, sliced
2 tbsp. mix berries
4 tsp. honey
1 tsp. chia seed
1 tsp. LSA mix

Directions

In a large bowl, mix all the cut fruits; add the chia seed and LSA mix. Toss well. Divide the ingredients in four parts and place in the middle of each wrap, then add 1 tsp. on top of each wrap. Gently fold at the ends, roll up, cut in half, and serve.

MEDITERRANEAN HERBED PASTA SALAD

Servings: 4

Ingredients

500 g pasta shells, cooked al dente
1 red capsicum
1 small bunch fresh basil, chopped
1 small bunch fresh Italian parsley, chopped
1 fresh celery stalk, thinly chopped
1 tbsp. fresh mint, chopped
250 g baby cherry tomatoes, sliced
1 fresh red chilli, chopped
1 fresh spring onion, chopped
1 clove garlic, chopped
2 tbsp. extra virgin olive oil
pinch sea salt (optional)
vinegar (optional)

Directions

Put the pasta in a serving dish. Add all remaining ingredients; toss very well and serve.

SWEET RICOTTA WRAP

Servings: 4

Ingredients

4 wraps
250 g fresh ricotta (drain the liquid)
1 tsp. vanilla essence
1 tbsp. sugar
1 tbsp. mixed dried citrus fruit (oranges, lemons, 99 percent fat free)
1 tbsp. chopped dark chocolate
1 tsp. chia seed
icing sugar for dusting

Directions

In a bowl, mix the ricotta with remaining ingredients (except the icing sugar). Toss very well, divide in four parts, and place in the middle of each wrap. Fold the ends, gently roll up, and cut in half. Dust each wrap with icing sugar and serve.

PIZZA WRAPS

Servings: 4

Ingredients

> 4 large wraps
> 4 fresh roma tomatoes, sliced
> 300 g mozzarella cheese, sliced
> ½ tsp. dried oregano
> ½ tsp. black pepper
> 4 pitted black olives, sliced
> 4 tsp. grated parmesan cheese
> 4 tsp. extra virgin olive oil

Directions

Place on top of the four wraps the mozzarella, tomatoes, olives, oregano, black pepper, 1 tsp. extra virgin olive oil, and 1 tsp. of grated parmesan. Fold the ends of each wrap, roll up, cut in half, and place on a non-stick pizza tray. Put in a preheated oven at 180° C for 10 minutes. Serve warm.

PASSIONFRUIT WRAPS

Servings: 4

Ingredients

4 wraps
4 fresh passion fruit, pulp drained
2 bananas, chopped
2 fresh mandarin oranges, chopped
1 tbsp. blueberry
1 tsp. chia seed
1 tsp. LSA mix
1 tsp. pistachios, chopped

Directions

Mix all the fruits in a bowl; then divide in four parts. Place in middle of each wrap, fold at the ends, roll up, and then cut in the middle and serve with your favourite ice cream.

EXOTIC FRUIT SALAD

Servings: 4

Ingredients

- 2 fresh mangos, sliced
- 2 bananas, sliced
- 2 papayas, sliced
- 2 passion fruit, chopped
- 2 kiwi fruit, sliced
- 2 tbsp. mix berries
- 50 g almonds, chopped
- 50 g pistachios, chopped
- 1 tbsp. mint, chopped
- 1 tsp. chia seed
- 1 tsp. LSA mix

Directions

Mix all ingredients in a large salad bowl; toss very well and serve.

SWEET WRAPS

Servings: 4

Ingredients

4 wraps
100 g dried prunes, chopped
100 g dried figs, chopped
100 g dried dates, chopped
100 g dried sultanas
100 g dried citrus peel (orange or lemon)
1 tsp. finely chopped almonds
1 tsp. finely chopped pistachios
1 tsp. finely chopped walnuts
4 tsp. golden syrup

Directions

Mix all the ingredients in a large bowl; toss very well, and then divide in four parts. Place in the middle of each wrap, then fold at the ends, roll up, cut in half, and serve.

MOZZARELLA CHEESE AND BOILED EGG WRAPS

Servings: 4

Ingredients

4 wraps
4 boiled eggs, chopped
1 large ball mozzarella cheese, sliced
4 fresh tomatoes, sliced
50 g fresh spinach, chopped
1 spring onion, chopped
1 clove garlic, chopped
1 small bunch fresh basil, chopped
1 tsp. chia seed
salt and pepper (optional)

Directions

In a large bowl, mix all the ingredients. Toss well and then divide in four parts. Place mixture in the middle of each wrap and then fold at the ends, roll up, and cut in half. Place on a non-stick tray and warm in 180° C oven for 5 minutes. Serve.

SUNSHINE WRAPS

Servings: 4

Ingredients

4 wraps
4 large roma tomatoes, chopped
200 g feta cheese, chopped
185 g tuna in oil, Italian style
1 small head lettuce, chopped
1 red capsicum, chopped
1 cucumber, chopped
1 celery stalk, chopped
4 pitted black olives, chopped
2 spring onions, chopped
1 tbsp. fresh basil, chopped
1 tbsp. fresh baby spinach, chopped
2 tbsp. fresh lemon juice
1 fresh red chilli, chopped
2 tbsp. extra virgin olive oil
1 tsp. chia seed
salt and pepper (optional)

Directions

In a large bowl, mix all fresh ingredients with feta and tuna. Toss very well and divide in four parts. Place evenly over the wraps, fold in half and then again and again. You should end up with cone-shaped wraps, ready to serve.

MEDITERRANEAN ANTIOXIDANT COUSCOUS

Servings: 1

Ingredients

500 g fresh tomato, chopped
500 g couscous
1/2 cup fresh parsley, finely chopped
1/2 cup fresh mint, finely chopped
juice of 6 fresh lemons
8 fresh spring onions, finely chopped
2 cloves garlic, finely chopped
4 tbsp. extra virgin olive oil
1 tbsp. premium cultured butter
1 cup hot water
1 small hot chilli, chopped
salt and pepper (optional)

Directions

Place 500 g couscous in a heatproof bowl. Add 1 cup boiling water. Add the butter; mix well and cover with lid for 2 minutes; then fluff up the couscous with a fork until no lumps are left. Add chopped tomato, chopped parsley, chopped spring onions, chopped garlic, chopped hot chilli, lemon juice, 4 tbsp. extra virgin olive oil, salt, and pepper. Mix very well and serve.

PUMPKIN GNOCCHI WITH RICOTTA CHEESE

Servings: 6

Ingredients

1.5 kg sliced pumpkin
100 g plain white flour
1 tsp. salt
1 tsp. butter
1 egg
100 g ricotta cheese
1 litre water for cooking
grated parmesan cheese (optional)

Directions

Preheat oven to 150° C. Place sliced pumpkin on a tray and put in oven for 15 minutes. Once pumpkin is cooked, puree the pulp. Place the puree in a pot, and stir while adding flour, egg, and salt. Pour water in a saucepan, add salt, and bring to a boil.

Using a teaspoon, make one scoop of the pumpkin at a time and drop into the boiling water. When the dumplings rise to the top of the water, remove and place on a plate. Add butter and ricotta cheese. Serve topped with grated parmesan cheese.

LASAGNE ITALIANA

Servings: 6

Ingredients

PASTA AND RED SAUCE

200 g lasagne sheets
600 g premium beef mince
785 g chunky tomato sauce
1 onion, chopped
2 cloves garlic, finely chopped
2 cups grated mozzarella cheese
3 tbsp. white wine (optional)
How olive oil
salt and black pepper (optional)

BECHAMEL SAUCE

2 cups milk
½ cup plain flour
60 g butter

Directions

Heat the oil in a pan. Add onion, garlic, and beef mince, and simmer for 1 minute. Then add white wine, tomato sauce, salt, and pepper, and simmer on low for 15-20 minutes.

For béchamel:

Melt butter in a separate saucepan. Add flour gradually to the butter, and stir until smooth. Add milk, and keep stirring until sauce thickens; then remove from heat.

Place the first layer of lasagne sheets in a deep, non-stick oven dish. Add a layer of sauce and mozzarella cheese. Repeat step until dish has room for one more layer. Cover the top layer with béchamel sauce and bake for 25 minutes or until golden brown.

MEDITERRANEAN GRILLED SALAD

Servings: 8

Ingredients

SALAD

    3 capsicums, cut in half (red, yellow, green)
    3 tomatoes, sliced
    2 zucchini, sliced
    2 spring onions, chopped
    2 eggplant, sliced
    200 g feta cheese

SALAD DRESSING

    50 g extra virgin olive oil
    2 tbsp. balsamic vinegar
    6 mint leaves
    6 basil leaves
    6 baby spinach leaves
    1 clove garlic, crushed
    salt and pepper

Directions

Place eggplant and zucchini onto a heated grill, and cook gently until golden brown, approximately 5 minutes per side. Grill the full capsicum 10 minutes on each side and then peel the skin. Place olive oil, vinegar, mint, basil, spinach, and garlic into a bowl and mix well. Place grilled eggplant, zucchini, and capsicum on a large platter.

Add dressing, salt, and pepper to taste, and mix well. Top with tomato, onion, and feta cheese. Serve with your favourite bread.

MEDITERRANEAN MINESTRONE SOUP

Servings: 6

Ingredients

300 g tomato, chopped
2 carrots, thinly sliced
2 celery sticks, chopped
2 garlic cloves, crushed
2 onions, chopped
2 large zucchini, sliced
2 large potatoes, sliced
200 g broccoli
200 g peas
2 tbsp. red lentils
2 tbsp. brown lentils
1 tbsp. dry vegetable stock
2 tbsp. extra virgin olive oil
6 cups water
salt and pepper (optional, to taste)

Directions

Place all ingredients in a saucepan, except extra virgin olive oil. Cover and bring to boil. Reduce heat and simmer for 45 minutes or until vegetables and lentils are tender. Add extra virgin olive oil and serve.

MIXED TONGUE SALAD

Ingredients

4 boiled large potatoes, sliced
1 large ball mozzarella, sliced
2 medium eggplant, grilled, sliced
4 large tomatoes, sliced
4 large boiled eggs, sliced
1 bunch spinach

Dressing

3 tbsp. olive oil
2 tbsp. balsamic vinegar
salt and pepper (optional)

Directions

Wash tomato and spinach very well. In a large, flat container, layer the spinach. On top, place the sliced tomato, potato, eggplant, mozzarella, and boiled egg. Top with dressing, and serve with your favourite bread.

MEDITERRANEAN BREAD SALAD

Servings: 6

Ingredients

1 kg fresh diced tomatoes
250 g mixed olives
1/2 cup fresh mint, chopped
2 cloves garlic, chopped
150 g feta cheese, cut in small pieces
6 fresh spring onions, chopped
12 slices bruschetta bread (whole-meal bread)
4 tbsp. extra virgin olive oil
1 hot chilli or pepper
pinch of oregano (optional)

Directions

Preheat oven to 180° C. Bake sliced bread for 5 to 10 minutes or until golden, then break into small chunks and keep cool in a salad bowl while you prepare all the other ingredients. In a salad bowl, combine tomato, mixed olives, mint, garlic, spring onions, hot chilli, extra virgin olive oil, and a pinch of oregano. Mix well with chunks of bread, and serve with feta cheese on top.

SARDINE RIPIENE (SARDINE SANDWICH)

Servings: 8

Ingredients

1 kg fresh sardine (clean and open)
300 g breadcrumbs
2 garlic cloves, finely chopped
3 tbsp. fresh parsley, chopped
1 tbsp. mint, chopped
3 tbsp. fresh lemon juice
2 tbsp. extra virgin olive oil
salt and pepper (optional)
extra oil for cooking

Directions

In a large bowl, mix very well breadcrumbs, garlic, parsley, mint, lemon juice, olive oil, salt and pepper. Take each of the clean, opened sardines and put on the open side 2 tbsp. of the mix ingredients, and put on top another sardine, like a sandwich. Place the sardine sandwich in a wide cook pot; season to taste on top with olive oil, salt, and pepper. Cover and simmer over medium heat for 10 or 12 minutes. Serve with lemon and fresh salad.

MARINATED PRAWNS WITH ITALIAN HERBS

Servings: 4

Ingredients

1 kg clean, fresh prawns
2 tbsp. fresh chopped parsley
1 tbsp. fresh mint, chopped
1 tbsp. fresh basil, chopped
2 fresh garlic cloves, finely crushed
5 tbsp. extra virgin olive oil
salt and pepper (optional)
8 wooden skewers

Directions

Put the prawns into a bowl. Add the garlic, parsley, mint, basil, olive oil, salt, and pepper. Stir all the ingredients together very well. Cover and chill in the refrigerator for 1 hour to marinate. Thread prawns onto wooden skewers; fry or grill for 5 minutes or until they are pink.

FRESH FISH WITH ONIONS, CAPERS, AND VINEGAR (SALMON, TROUT, SWORDFISH OR MULLET)

Servings: 4

Ingredients

1 kg fresh swordfish, trout, salmon, or mullet
2 cups plain flour
2 onions, chopped
2 tbsp. capers
3 tbsp. vinegar
4 tbsp. olive oil for frying
salt and pepper (optional)

Directions

After washing the fish, pat dry with paper towels. Put the flour in a plastic bag with pinch of salt and pepper, and add the fish. Seal the bag, and toss together so that the fish is well coated in the flour.

In a frying pan, heat oil. Fry the fish for 2 minutes on each side or till fish is crisp and golden. Place in a serving dish.

Heat the remaining oil in another pan. Fry onions and capers for 2 to 3 minutes until soft and golden; then splash in the vinegar, a pinch of salt and pepper. Turn off and cover for 1 minute, then put the cooked onion and capers on top the fish and serve.

LIGHT SUPPER OF APPLE AND PRAWN SALAD

Servings: 4

Ingredients

1 cup cooked rice
2 small red apples
1 green and 1 red pepper (remove core and seeds)
2 tomatoes
1 stalk celery
1 tbsp. fresh parsley, chopped
15 fresh peeled prawns
3 tbsp. extra virgin olive oil
2 tbsp. lemon juice
salt and pepper (optional)
4 scallop shells

Directions

In a bowl, mix together cold rice, skinned chopped tomatoes, diced apple, diced pepper, and chopped celery, oil and lemon juice, salt and pepper (optional). Mix well, and then pile in scallop shells. Top with prawns and garnish with chopped parsley and serve.

MOUSSAKA

Servings: 6

Ingredients

800 g eggplant
120 ml olive oil
2 medium onions, chopped
2 large tomatoes
500 g minced lamb
2 tbsp. tomato puree
2 tbsp. fresh parsley, chopped
1 tbsp. basil, chopped
3 tbsp. white wine
1 tsp. ground cinnamon
salt and pepper
4 tbsp. toasted breadcrumbs

For sauce:

50 g butter
50 g plain flour
600 ml milk
25 g grated parmesan cheese

Directions

To make white sauce: Melt the butter in a small pan, and stir in the flour. Heat while stirring for 1 minute. Remove from heat and gradually blend in the milk. Return to the heat, and cook, stirring, for 2 minutes until thickened. Add the nutmeg, parmesan cheese, salt, and pepper.

Cut eggplant slices 5 mm thick, and then layer them in a colander, sprinkling each layer with salt. Let stand for 20 minutes, and then remove the excess water and pat them dry on kitchen paper.

In a large frying pan, heat some oil and fry the eggplant until golden on both sides. Then let them dry on kitchen paper. Put the tomatoes into boiling water for 25 seconds, refresh in cold water, and peel the skins away and chop them.

Preheat oven 180° C/350° F

Heat 2 tbsp. oil in a frying pan. Add onions and minced lamb. Fry gently for 6 minutes, stirring and breaking up the minced lamb with a wooden spoon. Add the tomatoes, salt and pepper, cinnamon, parsley, tomato puree, and wine, and bring to boil. Reduce the heat, cover with a lid, and simmer for 14 to 15 minutes. Layer eggplant in shallow, ovenproof dish; add the minced meat, sauce, and then eggplant on top like lasagne. Make the white sauce and pour over the eggplant. Sprinkle with breadcrumbs and parmesan. Bake for 45 minutes or until golden.

EGGS WITH RICOTTA AND VEGETABLE

Servings: 4

Ingredients

1 onion, finely chopped
1 clove garlic, finely chopped
2 tbsp. olive oil
1/2 cauliflower, cut in small pieces
300 g pumpkin, cut in small pieces
2 medium potatoes, cut in small pieces
2 medium tomatoes, cut in small pieces
200 g peas
250 g fresh ricotta cheese
4 fresh eggs
1/2 cup water or vegetable stock
salt and pepper

Directions

Heat oil in a saucepan. Add onion and garlic. Cook until golden, and then add potato, cauliflower, pumpkin, peas, and tomato. Cook for 5 minutes, add water, cover, and cook for 10 minutes. Add ricotta on top of vegetables and then the eggs, salt and pepper. Cover and cook until eggs are firm. Serve hot.

RICE AND POTATO SOUP

Servings: 6

Ingredients

600 g potatoes chopped in small piece
150 g rice
1 onion finely, chopped
1 tbsp. fresh chopped parsley
2 tbsp. extra virgin olive oil
40 g cholesterol-free olive oil spread (canola)
1/2 cup parmesan cheese
salt and pepper

Directions

Heat half of the spread and 1 tbsp. olive oil in a saucepan. Add onion and potato; cook until golden. Add rice, salt, and pepper. Cover rice with water, and cook for 15 minutes or until rice is softer. When ready, add the rest of the spread and parmesan cheese. Serve with fresh parsley on top.

MUSSELS GRATINATE

Servings: 6-8

Ingredients

1,500 g mussels, very well cleaned
1 onion, finely chopped
2 cloves garlic, finely chopped
2 tbsp. fresh parsley, finely chopped
150 g breadcrumbs
40 g capers, finely chopped
1 lemon
3 fillets of anchovy, finely chopped
2 tbsp. extra virgin olive oil
salt and pepper

Directions

Place unopened mussels in a large pan—no water required. Cover and cook for 3 to 5 minutes. Give the pan a shake. Then start removing any opened mussels and set them aside. Heat oil in a frying pan; add garlic, onion, capers, anchovies, parsley, breadcrumbs, salt, and pepper. Cook until golden, and then remove from stove. Place 1 tbsp. of this mixture in each of the mussels and place in an oven dish. Cook in grill oven a few minutes until golden.

FAST FETTUCCINE

Servings: 4

Ingredients

500 g fettuccine
300 g mushrooms, washed and sliced
100 g prosciutto, cut in small pieces
1 clove garlic, chopped
12 fresh basil leaves, washed and chopped
2 tbsp. extra virgin olive oil
parmesan cheese
salt and pepper

Directions

Heat oil in a saucepan. Add garlic and mushrooms; cook for 5 minutes. Add prosciutto, basil, salt, and pepper. Cook for 5 minutes and then remove from stove.

Cook fettuccine by following package directions; then drain and mix with mushroom sauce. Serve with parmesan cheese on top.

QUICK TAGLIATELLE WITH TUNA

Servings: 4

Ingredients

500 g tagliatelle pasta
185 g can tuna
4 anchovies, cut small
2 cloves garlic, chopped
2 tbsp. extra virgin olive oil
salt and pepper

Directions

Heat oil in a frying pan. Add garlic, anchovies, tuna, salt, and pepper. Cook for 5 minutes and then remove from stove.

Cook tagliatelle pasta by following package directions; place with tuna sauce, mix well, and serve.

MEATBALL FRITTERS

Servings: 6

Ingredients

500 g minced meat
2 fresh eggs
50 g breadcrumbs
1 tbsp. parmesan cheese
1 cup béchamel sauce (recipe below)
1 clove garlic, finely chopped
1 tbsp. fresh parsley, chopped
salt and pepper

Ingredient for béchamel:

2 cups milk
½ cup plain flour
60 g butter

Directions

For béchamel sauce, melt butter in a saucepan. Add flour, gradually stirring gently until smooth. Gradually add milk and stir until sauce thickens. Remove from heat.

Place béchamel in a bowl. Add minced meat, eggs, parmesan cheese, garlic, parsley, salt, and pepper. Mix well, and then divide mixture into balls. Gently roll them in breadcrumbs, coating balls evenly. Dip fry until golden, and drain on paper towels. Serve hot.

SWEET PUMPKIN CHIPS

Ingredients

1 kg pumpkin
200 g plain flour
2 beaten eggs
150 g sugar
1 grated lemon rind
1 tsp. cinnamon powder
vegetable oil for frying
icing sugar
pinch of salt

Directions

Cut pumpkin, and cover with foil. Cook in oven until soft. When ready, place pulp into bowl. Add flour, eggs, sugar, grated lemon, cinnamon, and salt. Mix well until it forms a smooth dough. Then cut into chips, shape, and fry until golden and crisp. Place on a paper towel to drain oil before serving sprinkled with icing sugar.

RICE AND RICOTTA FRITTERS

Servings: 6-7

Ingredients

300 g rice
250 g fresh ricotta; drain excess water
3 beaten eggs
2 tbsp. parmesan cheese
1 clove garlic, finely chopped
1 tbsp. mint finely chopped
1 tbsp. parsley, finely chopped
200 g breadcrumbs
pinch of saffron
no-cholesterol vegetable oil for frying
salt and pepper

Directions

Cook rice with a pinch of saffron in salty, boiling water until tender. When ready, drain well and place in a bowl. Allow to cool, and then add ricotta, eggs, parmesan cheese, parsley, mint, garlic, salt, and pepper. Mix very well, and divide mixture into small balls, coating them evenly in breadcrumbs, and gently flatten.

Heat oil in a frying pan, and cook fritters until golden on each side. Drain on a paper towel and serve hot or cold.

TOMATO PARMIGIANA

Servings: 6-8

Ingredients

1 kg fresh tomatoes
150 g flour
3 fresh eggs, beaten
2 tbsp. parmesan cheese
300 g breadcrumbs
1 tbsp. fresh basil, finely chopped
1 tbsp. fresh parsley, finely chopped
1 clove garlic, finely chopped
olive oil
salt and pepper

Directions

In a container, combine breadcrumbs, parmesan cheese, basil, parsley, garlic, salt, and pepper. Wash and cut tomato slices. Dip in flour, then in eggs, and then in combined breadcrumbs. Fry in hot oil. Place on paper towels to drain. Serve hot.

QUICK ENERGY BOOSTER 1: BRUSCHETTA BREAD PIZZAIOLA

Ingredients

10 slices bruschetta bread
6 fresh tomato slices
10 slices fresh mozzarella cheese
10 black olives, sliced
3 tbsp. extra virgin olive oil
pinch of oregano
salt and pepper

Directions

Place bruschetta bread on grill tray. Cook both sides until golden, then place mozzarella on top of bread, followed by tomato, olive, pinch of oregano, olive oil, salt, and pepper. Return bread to the grill. Cook until bread is brown. Serve hot or cold.

QUICK ENERGY BOOSTER 2: BRUSCHETTA BREAD WITH TOMATO AND BASIL

Ingredients

10 slices bruschetta bread
6 fresh medium tomatoes, chopped in small pieces
12 fresh basil leaves, finely chopped
1 clove garlic, finely chopped
1 tbsp. extra virgin olive oil
pinch of oregano
salt and pepper

Directions

Place bruschetta bread in grill tray. Cook both sides until golden and set aside. In a bowl, combine tomato, basil, garlic, olive oil, oregano, salt, and pepper, and mix well. Top the bruschetta bread with the tomato mixture, and return to the grill until the bread is brown. serve hot or cold.

QUICK ENERGY BOOSTER 3: BRUSCHETTA BREAD WITH MUSHROOMS, TOMATO, AND ONIONS

Ingredients

10 slices bruschetta bread
10 mushrooms, sliced
1 onion, finely sliced
1 cup chunky tomato sauce
1 tbsp. extra virgin olive oil
salt and pepper

Directions

Place bruschetta bread on grill tray. Heat both sides until golden, and set aside. Heat oil in a frying pan; add onions and mushrooms, and cook for 5 minutes or until golden. Then add tomato, salt, and pepper. Toss and cook for 5 minutes. Top the bruschetta bread with this mixture, and return to the grill until bread is brown. Serve hot or cold.

GREEK SALAD

Ingredients

1 large head lettuce, washed and sliced
6 fresh tomatoes, sliced
100 g black and green olives
2 cucumbers, sliced
6 fresh spring onions, chopped
250 g feta cheese, crumbled

For dressing

5 tbsp. extra virgin olive oil
2 tbsp. fresh lemon juice
salt and pepper

Directions

In a large bowl, mix all the salad ingredients. Add oil, lemon juice, salt, and pepper. Mix well, and finish with extra feta cheese and black olives on top.

ITALIAN STUFFED SQUID

Ingredients

6 fresh squid
1 kg chopped tomato
3 tbsp. chopped parsley
2 cloves garlic, chopped
2 onions, chopped
50 g breadcrumbs
4 tbsp. olive oil
4 tbsp. white wine
2 tbsp. Parmesan cheese
salt and pepper

Directions

Wash and clean squid tubes and set aside. Clean and cut the rest of the squid in very small pieces.

For stuffing mixture:

Heat 2 tbsp. oil in a frying pan. Add the small-cut pieces of squid, 1 clove chopped garlic, 1 chopped onion, and parsley. Cook until onion is golden and then add wine. Cover and heat for 15 minutes. Add breadcrumbs, parmesan cheese, salt, and pepper. Stir well, and remove from stove.

Fill the squid tubes with the stuffing mixture. Secure the ends of the tubes with wooden cocktail sticks.

Heat 2 tbsp. oil in a deep frying pan. Add 1 clove chopped garlic, 1 chopped onion, and the stuffed squid, and fry until golden. Then add tomato, salt, and pepper. Cover and heat gently for 20 minutes.

ORECCHIETTI WITH BROCCOLI AND CAULIFLOWER

Servings: 8

Ingredients

    250 g white plain flour
    250 g plain wholemeal flour
    400 ml water
    300 g fresh broccoli
    200 g fresh cauliflower
    3 medium potatoes, boiled and cut in pieces
    1 onion, chopped
    2 garlic cloves, chopped
    160 g pancetta or capocollo, sliced and chopped
    1/2 cup fresh parsley, chopped
    1/2 cup fresh grated parmesan cheese
    3 tbsp. extra virgin olive oil
    2 fresh red hot chillies, chopped
    4 fillets of anchovy
    salt and pepper

Directions

In a bowl, place flour, water, and pinch of salt. Mix to a smooth dough and then place the same flour on a flat surface and roll the dough into a 2-cm cylinder. Cut into 2-cm lengths, using flour press and flatten each with your finger. Gently roll a small knife to each piece. Make the shape of orecchietti (little ears); place them on a floured container until ready to cook.

In a large pan of salted, boiling water, add broccoli, cauliflower, and orecchietti. Cook until broccoli is tender.

Heat oil in a frying pan. Add onion, garlic, pancetta, anchovies, hot chillies, potatoes, and parsley. Cook gently until golden. With slotted spoon, remove from water broccoli, cauliflower, and orecchietti and place into the frying pan. Toss and cook for half minutes. Add parmesan cheese, salt, and pepper. Mix well, add a bit of the broccoli water if needed, and then remove from stove. Serve hot.

SPAGHETTI WITH AGLIO E OLIO

Servings: 4-5

Ingredients

500 g spaghetti
4 cloves garlic, finely chopped
4 tbsp. extra virgin olive oil
2 hot chillies, finely chopped
40 g dry breadcrumbs
3 tbsp. parmesan cheese
salt and pepper

Directions

Cook spaghetti in salted, boiling water until al dente. Heat oil in a large frying pan. Add garlic and hot chillies, and cook gently until golden. Add breadcrumbs, salt, and pepper. Stir well, and remove from stove. When pasta is al dente, drain and toss in the pan with parmesan cheese. Serve hot.

STUFFED PEPPERS WITH ANTIOXIDANT COUSCOUS

Servings: 10

Ingredients

10 bell peppers
500 g packed couscous
2 cups hot water
1/2 cup fresh parsley, finely chopped
1/2 cup fresh mint, finely chopped
juice of 6 fresh lemons
8 fresh spring onions, finely chopped
2 cloves garlic, finely chopped
4 tbsp. extra virgin olive oil
1 small hot chilli, chopped
400 g fresh tomato, chopped
salt and pepper

Directions

Cut off the top of each pepper, and remove the core and seeds. Place couscous in a large bowl; add hot water and salt. Stir and let sit for 5 minutes. Then add parsley, mint, spring onions, garlic, hot chilli, tomato, lemon juice, and the extra virgin olive oil, salt, and pepper. Mix very well.

Using a spoon, fill the peppers with the couscous mixture. Place them in an oiled, ovenproof dish, and bake for 20 minutes or until tender.

TOMATOES STUFFED WITH RICE

Servings: 4

Ingredients

    4 large, ripe tomatoes
    150 g rice, boiled
    2 cloves garlic, chopped
    2 onions, chopped
    100 g tomato pulp, chopped
    2 tbsp. olive oil
    3 tbsp. grated parmesan cheese
    salt and pepper

Directions

Cut the tops off of tomatoes; scoop out the pulp and seeds using a teaspoon. Chop tomato pulp and set aside.

Heat olive oil in a large frying pan. Add garlic and onions. Cook until golden, and then add tomato pulp, salt, and pepper, and cook for 5 minutes. Add boiled rice and parmesan cheese, and simmer for 5 minutes.

Spoon mixture into the tomatoes, and bake uncovered for 20 minutes or until golden.

OCTOPUS, POTATO, AND ONION STEW

Servings: 6

Ingredients

1 kg baby octopus, cleaned and washed
2 large onions, chopped
2 cloves garlic, chopped
4 large potatoes, chopped
2 tbsp. fresh parsley, chopped
150 ml red wine
300 g chopped tomatoes
1/2 cup water
salt and pepper

Directions

Heat oil in a saucepan. Add onions, garlic, baby octopus, and parsley. Fry until golden, then add wine. Cover and cook for 5 minutes. Add tomato, potato, a half cup of water, salt, and pepper. Stir and cover. Cook for 20 minutes or until octopus is tender and sauce thickened.

OCTOPUS SALAD

Servings: 4

Ingredients

1 kg fresh, cleaned octopus
1/2 cup fresh parsley, chopped
1/2 cup fresh mint, chopped
2 cloves garlic, chopped
1 hot red chilli, chopped
juice of 1 fresh lemon
4 tbsp. extra virgin olive oil
salt and pepper

Directions

Place octopus in a large pan with boiling water. Boil for 1 hour or until tender. Using a sharp knife, cut octopus into bite-size pieces. Place in salad container; add parsley, mint, garlic, hot chilli, lemon juice, olive oil, salt, and pepper. Mix well and serve.

BLACK OLIVE BREAD

Ingredients for dough

470 g plain flour
25 g fresh baker's yeast, in 1/2 cup warm water
400 ml warm water
2 tbsp. olive oil
salt

Extra ingredients:

250 g pitted black olives
250 g semi-dry tomato, finely chopped
2 tbsp. fresh parsley, chopped
2 tbsp. chopped fresh mint, chopped

Directions

To make the pizza dough, dissolve fresh yeast in 1/2 cup warm water. Stir until dissolved. Put the flour on a flat surface. Make a well in the centre, add the dissolved yeast, salt, 2 tbsp. olive oil, and combine well. Pour in warm water, bit by bit, and mix well with your hand until it forms sticky dough. Add more flour and knead for a few minutes until the dough is soft, elastic, and smooth. Sprinkle the dough with flour. Cover with cling wrap first and a tablecloth. Keep warm and allow to rise for one and a half hours or until doubled in size.

When dough is ready, turn onto a floured surface. Add the extra ingredients: black olive, dry tomato, parsley, and mint, and mix well. Knead for about 5 minutes, and then cut in half and shape into two rounds. Place on two lightly greased baking trays, cover with lightly oiled cling wrap. Keep warm and allow to rise for 1 hour or until doubled in size.

Preheat oven to 220° C. After the dough is ready, slash the tops with a knife, and then bake for about 40 minutes or until top and bottom are golden brown.

HOW TO PRESERVE FRESH TOMATOES

What You Need

box with fresh tomatoes
clean jugs or glass bottles with lids
salt and fresh basil (optional)
big container or big pan to boil the jugs

Preserve Tomatoes with Skin

Wash the tomatoes, cut into pieces, and put them into the big bucket. Mix with salt, after they are ready to put into the jugs, and secure the lid properly. Put them inside the big pan or cooking container. Fill up with water, and boil for 30 minutes.

After the water cools down, pull them out and dry them with a clean cloth. Now they are ready to store for up to two or three years.

Preserve without Skin

Put boiling water into the sink, and put in the whole, clean tomato (uncut). Let them sit in the hot water for ten minutes. Take them out with a sieve if manageable. You can start to peel the skin off and put the tomatoes into the jugs. Secure the top lid and put in a pan. Fill the pan with cold water, and boil for 30 minutes. When cooled down, dry the jugs and save for storage for as long as you like.

DATE AND ZUCCHINI LOAF

Makes 3 loaves

Ingredients

6 eggs
2 cups canola or vegetable oil
2 cups brown sugar
2 capfuls vanilla essence
Approx 2 cups milk
2 zucchini, grated
2 cups chopped dates (soaked overnight)
7 cups sifted flour
3 tsp. cinnamon

Directions

Beat eggs, sugar, oil and, vanilla essence in a large bowl until creamy. Slowly add flour, dates and zucchini, and then 2 cups milk. Combine all together with spoon until well mixed; then spoon into loaf tins lined with baking paper, and bake approx 3/4 hour at 175° C.

PUMPKIN SOUP WITH BUTTERED BREAD

Ingredients

oil
2 cloves garlic
4 onions
1 large pumpkin
6 carrots
16 potatoes
8 tsp. Vegeta
3-3/4 cups rice (cook before placing in soup)

Directions

Sauté garlic and onion in oil, and then add all the vegetables and Vegeta. Add enough water to cover, and allow to cook. When cooked, puree, and then add the cooked rice.

MEDITERRANEAN GRILLED SALAD

Servings: 6-8

Ingredients

3 capsicums (red, yellow, green), cut in half
3 tomatoes, sliced
2 zucchini, sliced
2 spring onion, chopped
2 eggplant, sliced
200 g feta cheese

For dressing

50 g extra virgin olive oil
2 tbsp. balsamic vinegar
6 mint leaves
6 basil leaves
6 baby spinach leaves
1 clove garlic, crushed
salt and pepper

Directions

Place sliced eggplant and zucchini onto a heated grill. Heat slowly until golden brown. Grill the capsicum and peel the skin. Put olive oil, vinegar, mint, basil, spinach, and garlic into a bowl and mix well. On a large platter, put the grilled eggplant, zucchini, and capsicum. Add the dressing, salt, and pepper, and mix well. Then, on top, place tomato, onion, and feta cheese. Serve with your favourite bred.

SPAGHETTI NAPOLETANA

Servings: 4-5

Ingredients

2 tbsp. extra virgin olive oil
2 garlic cloves, chopped
1 large onion, chopped
2 tbsp. basil, chopped
1 tbsp. black olive, sliced
500 g tomato, chopped
400 g spaghetti
parmesan cheese
salt and pepper
1 tsp. sugar

Directions

Place oil, garlic, and onion in a frying pan; heat gently for 2 minutes. Add black olive and basil, and simmer for 1 minute. Then add tomato, salt and pepper, and 1 teaspoon sugar. Heat on low for 10 or 15 minutes or until slightly thickened. Cook spaghetti al dente or according to the instructions on the package; then drain well and serve with Napolitano sauce and parmesan cheese on top.

SPAGHETTI WITH BLACK SAUCE OF CUTTLEFISH AND PEAS

Servings: 6

Ingredients

500 g spaghetti
500 g fresh cuttlefish with ink
300 g peas
700 g tomato sauce
1 small onion
2 garlic cloves
2 tbsp. parsley, chopped
3 tbsp. olive oil
1 cup water
2 tsp. sugar
salt and pepper

Directions

Gently cut the top middle of the cuttlefish. Carefully take the black ink bag and place it in a half cup of water. Open the bag with fork or knife, and let the ink mix with water and set aside. Then clean, wash, and cut cuttlefish.

In a saucepan, slowly heat olive oil add chopped onion, garlic, and parsley. Stir for 1 minute and then add the cuttlefish. Simmer for 3 minutes. Spray with white wine if you like. Cover and cook on low for 5 minutes. Add peas, tomato, 1/2 cup of water, sugar, salt, and black pepper. Simmer for a few seconds and then add the black ink. Cover and cook gently for 45 minutes or until sauce thickens.

Cook spaghetti in salted boiling water by following package directions, then drain well and serve with the black sauce and cuttlefish on top.

SPAGHETTI WITH FRIED ZUCCHINI

Ingredients

Olive oil or no-cholesterol sunflower oil
500 g spaghetti
500 g zucchini, sliced
2 garlic cloves
100 g pecorino romano or parmesan cheese
salt and black pepper

Directions

Heat the sunflower oil in a frying pan, and fry the zucchini with a pinch of salt. When they turn golden, flip and fry the other side. When ready, remove and place zucchini in a dish to keep warm while you cook the spaghetti in salted boiling water. When it is cooked al dente or according to the instructions on the package, drain well and put spaghetti on a warmed plate. Fry the garlic in the same oil left from the zucchini, and then add spaghetti and zucchini, pinch of salt, and black pepper. Remove from stove and sprinkle with pecorino or parmesan cheese. Serve at once.

PASTA AL FORNO (BAKED IN OVEN)

Ingredients

500 g macaroni pasta
800 g tomato sauce
300 g lean minced meat
200 g peas
2 eggplant, sliced and grilled
1 onion, chopped
2 cloves garlic, chopped
3 beaten eggs
60 g parmesan cheese
3 tbsp. olive oil
salt and pepper
white wine (optional)

Directions

Prepare the mince sauce by heating oil in a saucepan. Add onion, garlic, then minced meat. Simmer gently for 2 minutes. Add 3 tbsp. wine; cover and simmer for 3 minutes. Add peas, tomato sauce, salt, and pepper. Cover and cook for 20 minutes or until sauce thickens. Cook pasta in salted boiling water by following instructions on package. When ready, drain pasta well, and put it in a large bowl. Add the mince sauce, grilled and sliced eggplant, parmesan cheese, beaten eggs, salt, and pepper. Mix well. Have an oven dish ready, battered and sprinkled with breadcrumbs on bottom and sides to prevent sticking. Place pasta and sauce with all the ingredients; sprinkle with more parmesan cheese on top. Bake at 170° C for 20 minutes or until the top is golden. When ready, remove from oven and let rest for 15 minutes before serving.

TAGLIATELLE ALLA SICILIANA

Servings: 4-5

Ingredients

500 g Italian continental sausage
1 large eggplant, cut in thin strips
1 clove garlic, chopped
1 onion, chopped
1 tbsp. olive oil
500 g tagliatelle pasta
parmesan cheese
salt and pepper
2 tbsp. white wine

Directions

Heat oil in a medium saucepan. Add onion, garlic, and Italian sausage. Cover and cook for 5 minutes, and then flip the sausage and add the wine. Cover and simmer gently for 5 minutes, then remove sausage from saucepan and add eggplant. Cover and simmer for 2 minutes. Chop the sausage and put back in saucepan. Mix well with the eggplant, and simmer for 5 minutes. Add salt and pepper, and remove from stove.

Cook tagliatelle following package directions; drain and place into saucepan with the sausage and eggplant. Mix together and serve with parmesan cheese.

SPAGHETTINI WITH EGGPLANT AND TOMATO SAUCE

Servings: 6

Ingredients:

l kg tomato, chopped
4 eggplant, sliced thin
1 onion, chopped
100 g grated parmesan cheese
10 fresh basil leaves
1 clove garlic, chopped
2 tbsp. extra virgin olive oil
no-cholesterol sunflower oil (for frying eggplant)
salt and pepper

Directions

Place eggplant in a colander. Sprinkle every layer with salt, and let rest for 20 minutes. Heat the olive oil in a pan. Add onions and garlic, and cook until golden. Add the chopped tomato, basil, salt, and pepper. Simmer gently for 45 minutes or until sauce thickens.

After 20 minutes, squeeze the juice out of the eggplant and drain them with paper towels. Heat the oil in a pan, and fry the eggplant on each side until golden. Dry excess oil, and cut them into long strips. In the meantime, cook spaghettini in salted boiling water following package directions. Drain spaghettini and toss with tomato sauce; add eggplant. Mix well, and serve with parmesan cheese on top.

SICILIAN POTATO CAKES

Servings: 6

Ingredients

1 kg potatoes
3 eggs, lightly beaten
3 tbsp. fresh parsley, chopped
2 garlic cloves, finely chopped
50 g grated parmesan cheese
150 g breadcrumbs
60ml. olive oil or no-cholesterol sunflower oil
salt and black pepper (and plain flour optional)

Directions

Wash and put potatoes in a large pan. Cover with water, and boil until soft.

When the potatoes are ready, drain and peel the skin; then place into a bowl and mash. Add parsley, garlic, parmesan cheese, breadcrumbs, eggs, salt, and pepper. Cover and chill for 45 minutes; then divide the potato mixture into balls and gently flatten. Place them in a large dish. (Dredge with plain flour if you like.) Heat the oil in a frying pan, and fry the potato cakes until golden brown on each side. Drain on paper towels and serve hot or cold with your favourite salad.

MACARONI SIRACUSA

Servings: 6

Ingredients

2 tbsp. olive oil
5 peeled tomatoes, chopped
2 cloves garlic, chopped
1 eggplant, chopped
8 fresh basil leaves
2 grilled capsicum, thin slices (peel the skin off and clean the inside)
20 g capers
3 anchovy fillets
500 g macaroni
3 tbsp. parmesan cheese
salt and pepper

Directions

Heat oil in a saucepan. Add garlic, then tomato, basil, eggplant, grilled capsicum, capers, anchovy, salt, and pepper. Simmer gently for 15 minutes or until sauce thickens. Cook macaroni in salted boiling water, following package directions, then drain well and put into the saucepan. Mix well with sauce and add parmesan cheese on top.

PASTA CAPRICCOSA

Servings: 6

Ingredients:

500 g pasta ditali
1 kg fresh tomatoes, chopped
10 fresh basil leaves, chopped
100 g salty ricotta cheese
2 cloves garlic, chopped
1 hot chilli, chopped
3 tbsp. extra virgin olive oil
salt

Directions

Wash and chop tomato; combine with basil, garlic, and hot chilli. Place them in a large dish. Add salty ricotta and olive oil; mix well, and let rest for 30 minutes. Cook the ditali pasta in salted boiling water until al dente, or follow package directions. When ready, drain pasta and place with tomato and ricotta. Mix all the ingredients very well and serve.

MEDITERRANEAN RISOTTO

Servings: 6

Ingredients

3 tbsp. extra virgin olive oil
2 cups short rice (arborio)
1 onion, chopped
1 clove garlic, chopped
150 g broccoli, chopped
1 carrot, chopped
160 g peas
150 g pumpkin
1 tbsp. fresh mint, chopped
1 tbsp. fresh parsley, chopped
4 cups boiling chicken stock
2 tbsp. parmesan cheese
pepper

Directions

Heat oil in saucepan. Add garlic, onion, and rice. Cook for 1 minute. Add the chicken stock and bring to boil, then reduce heat, cover, and simmer gently for 10 or 15 minutes. Add vegetables, and cook for 7 minutes or until softened. When ready, stir in pepper, parmesan cheese, parsley, and mint.

MEDITERRANEAN EGGS

Servings: 6

Ingredients

2 eggplant, sliced
500 g fresh tomato, peeled and sliced
1 onion, sliced
2 cloves garlic, chopped
1 green capsicum, thin sliced
1 red capsicum, thin sliced
1 tbsp. fresh basil, chopped
4 tbsp. fresh parsley
2 tbsp. extra virgin olive oil
6 eggs
salt and pepper

Directions

Slice eggplant and sprinkle each side with salt. Let rest for 15 minutes. After squeezing the juice out of the eggplant and patting dry, heat oil in frying pan. Cook each side until golden. Add in some oil, onion, garlic, and basil. Simmer for 1 minute. Transfer to a shallow oven dish, and add chopped tomato, capsicum, salt, and pepper. Cover and cook in ready warm oven for 20 minutes. Break each egg into a cup. Make 6 hollows in the veggies and slide eggs in. Cover and bake for another 5 minutes or until eggs are firm. Sprinkle with fresh parsley before serving.

SPAGHETTI WITH MEATBALL SAUCE

Servings: 6

Ingredients

500 g peeled, chopped tomatoes
300 g lean minced meat (beef)
1 onion, chopped
2 cloves garlic, chopped
1 tbsp. basil, chopped
2 tbsp. olive oil
pinch of sugar
1 tbsp. fresh parsley, chopped
3 tbsp. parmesan cheese
2 fresh eggs
50 g breadcrumbs
salt and pepper

Directions

Prepare meatballs by placing minced beef in a bowl. Add fresh parsley, 1 chopped garlic clove, 2 fresh eggs, breadcrumbs, 1 tbsp. parmesan cheese, salt, and pepper. Mix very well and then shape the mixture into small balls, and place in a large dish.

Prepare the sauce by heating olive oil in a saucepan. Add onion, garlic, basil, tomato, pinch of sugar, salt, and pepper. Cover and cook gently for 15 minutes; then add meatballs in sauce. Cover and cook for another 15 minutes more or until meatball and sauce are ready.

Cook spaghetti in salted boiling water by following package directions. Then drain, place them on a serving plate. Add meatball sauce on top, and sprinkle with parmesan cheese and pepper to finish.

Ortensia Greco-Conte

TAGLIATELLE ALLA SICILIANA

Servings: 4-5

Ingredients

500 g Italian continental sausage
1 large eggplant, cut in thin strips
1 clove garlic, chopped
1 onion, chopped
1 tbsp. olive oil
500 g tagliatelle pasta
3 tbsp. parmesan cheese
2 tbsp. white wine
salt and pepper

Directions

Heat oil in a medium saucepan. Add onion, garlic, and Italian sausage. Cover and cook for 5 minutes; then turn the sausage to the other side and add the wine. Cover and simmer gently for 10 minutes, then remove sausage from saucepan and add eggplant. Cover and simmer for 2 minutes. Chop the sausage and put back in saucepan. Mix well with the eggplant, and simmer for 7 minutes. Add salt and pepper. Remove from stove.

Cook tagliatelle following package directions, then drain and place into saucepan with the sausage and eggplant. Mix together and serve with parmesan cheese and pepper on top.

SPAGHETTI WITH PRAWNS

Servings: 4

Ingredients

500 g spaghetti
1 onion, chopped
1 clove garlic, chopped
1 tbsp. fresh celery, chopped
500 g fresh, cleaned prawns
4 fresh, peeled tomatoes, chopped
1 hot chilli, chopped
1 tbsp. fresh parsley
2 tbsp. extra virgin olive oil
1 tbsp. white wine
salt and pepper

Directions

Heat olive oil in saucepan. Add garlic, onion, celery, parsley, hot chilli, and prawns. Cook for 1 minute, then spray with wine. Simmer for 1 minute, add tomato, salt, and pepper. Cover and cook for 10 minutes.

Cook spaghetti in salted boiling water for 9 minutes uncovered, following package directions, then drain and place in the prawn sauce. Mix well and serve with parmesan cheese on top.

MEDITERRANEAN BREAD SALAD

Servings: 6

Ingredients

1 kg fresh tomatoes, diced
250 g mixed olives
1/2 cup fresh mint, chopped
2 cloves garlic, chopped
150 g feta cheese, cut in small pieces
6 fresh spring onions, chopped
12 slices bruschetta bread (whole-meal bread)
4 tbsp. extra virgin olive oil
1 hot chilli or pepper
pinch of oregano

Directions

Preheat oven to 180° C. Bake sliced bread for 10 minutes until golden, then break into small chunks and keep cool in a salad bowl while you prepare all the other ingredients. Add to the salad bowl tomato, olives, mint, garlic, spring onions, hot chilli, olive oil, and pinch of oregano. Mix well with chunks bread, and serve with feta cheese on top.

MEDITERRANEAN FRITTATA

Servings: 8

Ingredients

8 fresh eggs, lightly beaten
10 fresh spinach leaves
1 large onion, sliced
2 cloves garlic, chopped
1 large potato, thinly sliced
2 zucchini, thinly sliced
4 mushrooms, thinly sliced
2 tbsp. fresh parsley, chopped
2 tbsp. olive oil
1 tbsp. parmesan cheese
1 tbsp. bread crumbs
salt and pepper

Directions

In a large, nonstick frying pan, heat the oil. Add garlic and onion and cook for 1 minute. Add thinly cut potato and cook for 7 minutes or until tender. Then add zucchini, mushrooms, spinach, salt, and pepper. Mix well and cook gently for 6 minutes.

In a bowl, combine beaten eggs, parmesan cheese, fresh parsley, and breadcrumbs. Mix well; then pour over the ingredients in frying pan. Cook gently until the eggs are set on the bottom.

To set the top, place frying pan under a preheated grill until firm and golden. When ready, turn out, and cut into wedges. Serve with your favourite salad.

CANNELLONI WITH RICOTTA AND SPINACH

(Optional sauce) Bolognese or tomato

Servings: 6

Ingredients

400 g instant, ready-dried cannelloni tubes or
375 g fresh lasagne sheets
2 bunches spinach (optional)
2 eggs, beaten
600 g fresh ricotta cheese
salt and pepper
parmesan cheese
breadcrumbs

Ingredients for bolognese sauce

500 g lean beef mince meat
1 onion, chopped
1 clove garlic, chopped
1 carrot, chopped
1 celery stick, chopped
1 tbsp. parsley, chopped
2 tbsp. white wine
700 g chunky tomato sauce
2 tsp. sugar
2 tbsp. olive oil
parmesan cheese, grated
salt and pepper

Ingredients for tomato sauce

700 g chunky tomato sauce
1 clove garlic, chopped
1 onion, chopped
1 tbsp. fresh basil, chopped
2 tbsp. olive oil
2 tsp. sugar
parmesan cheese, grated
salt and pepper

Directions

If using fresh lasagne sheets, place 2 sheets at a time in a large pan of boiling salted water. Cook about 2 minutes or until softened, then remove carefully and lay out flat on a large tray. Repeat the process with the remaining pasta sheets. Wash and steam spinach for 5 minutes. When ready, drain very well in colander. Place spinach in a bowl. Add ricotta, eggs, salt, and pepper. Mix well and set aside.

To make bolognese sauce

Heat oil in a saucepan. Add onion, garlic, carrot, celery, and parsley. Cook until golden. Add mince meat; cook for 5 minutes, stirring well until brown. Add wine and let evaporate. Add tomato, sugar, salt, and pepper. Cook for 15 minutes or until sauce is slightly thickened.

Continue next page . . .

Ortensia Greco-Conte

To make tomato sauce

Heat oil in a saucepan. Add onion and garlic; cook until golden, then add tomato, basil, sugar, salt, and pepper. Cook for 15 minutes or until sauce is slightly thickened.

Prepare ovenproof dish by greasing the bottom and sides. Sprinkle with breadcrumbs, then add 4 tbsp. tomato sauce. Layer the first lasagne sheets, and spoon 2 tbsp. of the spinach mix. Roll up seam-side-down in the ovenproof dish; repeat with the remaining lasagne and spinach mixture, forming one layer. Add on top the remaining tomato sauce and parmesan cheese. Bake for 30 minutes or until golden brown.

If using instant, dried cannelloni pasta tube instead, just fill the tube with spinach mixture and arrange in the oven dish. Add sauce and cheese, and bake for 30 minutes.

TAGLIATELLE PRIMAVERA

Servings: 6

Ingredients

500 g tagliatelle pasta
1 medium carrot, cut into strips
1 medium zucchini, cut into strips
6 medium mushrooms, thinly sliced
4 spring onions, chopped very small
1 tbsp. fresh parsley, chopped very small
1 tbsp. fresh basil, chopped very small
2 tbsp. tomato sauce
1 clove garlic, chopped
1/2 cup light cream
2 tbsp. extra virgin olive oil
salt and pepper

Directions

Cook tagliatelle in salted boiling water for 10 minutes or by following the package directions. When ready, drain well and put in a container.

Heat oil in a large pan. Add garlic and spring onions, and cook until golden. Then add carrot, zucchini, mushroom, parsley, and basil. Cover and cook gently for 6 minutes; add tomato sauce, salt, and pepper. Cover and cook for 5 minutes, then add cream and cook gently for 5 minutes or until sauce is slightly thickened. When sauce is ready, add tagliatelle. Mix very well, and remove from stove. Serve with fresh parmesan cheese on top.

SALMON POTATO CAKES

Servings: 6

Ingredients

1 kg potatoes, peeled, boiled, and mashed
250 g fresh or canned pink salmon
150 g breadcrumbs
3 eggs, lightly beaten
3 tbsp. fresh parsley, finely chopped
4 fresh spring onions, finely chopped
60 ml olive oil or no-cholesterol sunflower oil
1 clove garlic, finely chopped
2 tbsp. fresh mint, finely chopped
50 g grated parmesan cheese
plain flour
salt and pepper

Directions

Combine mashed potato, salmon, breadcrumbs, eggs, parsley, onions, garlic, mint, parmesan cheese, salt, and pepper in a bowl. Mix well and shape mixture into balls. Gently flatten and dredge with flour.

Heat oil in a nonstick frying pan, and cook cakes until golden brown on each side. Then drain on paper towels. Serve hot or cold with your favourite salad in dinner rolls.

FETTUCCINE CARBONARA

Servings: 4

Ingredients

6 slices Virginia ham, cut into thin strips
1/2 cup light cream
50 g grated parmesan cheese
350 g fettuccine pasta
2 eggs, lightly beaten
2 tbsp. olive oil
salt and pepper

Directions

Heat oil in a large frying pan. Add ham, and cook until golden; then remove from stove. In the meantime, cook pasta in boiling salted water for 10 minutes until al dente or by following the package directions. Then drain well and put in the pan with ham. Add eggs, cream, parmesan cheese, salt, and pepper. Toss well and return to stove. Cook on very low heat for about 1 minute or until sauce is slightly thickened. Remove from stove, and serve with fresh grated parmesan cheese and pepper on top.

CONCHIGLIONI WITH SPINACH AND RICOTTA

Servings: 6

Ingredients

300 g conchiglioni pasta
400 g chunky tomato sauce
500 g fresh ricotta
1 bunch fresh spinach
1 clove garlic, chopped
1 onion, finely chopped
2 tbsp. fresh basil, chopped
2 tbsp. olive oil
2 tsp. sugar
fresh parmesan cheese, grated
salt and pepper

Directions

Cook pasta in boiling salted water for 13 minutes or by following package directions. When ready, drain well and let cool in a large dish.

Wash and steam spinach for 3 minutes. When ready, drain very well and place in a bowl. Add ricotta, salt, and pepper. Mix well and set aside.

Heat oil in a saucepan. Add onion and garlic; cook until golden. Then add tomato, basil, sugar, salt, and pepper. Cook for 15 minutes. When ready, put the sauce in a large oven dish, and start to fill each pasta conchiglioni with the spinach mixture. Layer sauce on top; continue until the oven dish is full, then sprinkle the top with parmesan cheese and cook in ready warm oven for 10 minutes or until the cheese on top is golden.

HEALTHY VEGETABLES WITH COUSCOUS

Servings: 6

Ingredients

2 cups instant couscous
1 cup vegetable stock
1 cup skim milk
1 medium sweet potato, peeled and diced
1 medium eggplant, cut into strips
300 g pumpkin, peeled and diced
300 g baby beans
4 carrots, cut into strips
200 g fresh mushrooms
3 tbsp. extra virgin olive oil
salt and pepper

Directions

Wash and cut all the vegetables. Place onto baking trays. Add olive oil, salt, and pepper. Mix very well and bake at 200° C for 25 minutes.

In a saucepan, bring stock and milk to a boil, then remove from stove. Arrange couscous in a large dish. Add stock and milk and cover. After 5 minutes, fluff up couscous with a fork. Add on top of the healthy, colourful baked vegetables.

CAPONATA SICILIANA

This recipe can be used for storage.

Servings: 6

Ingredients

3 medium eggplants, washed and diced
3 celery stalks, chopped
1 onion, chopped
2 cloves garlic, chopped
50 g capers
8 green olives, sliced
8 black olives, sliced
3 tbsp. tomato sauce
1 tbsp. sugar
1 tbsp. vinegar
olive oil
salt and pepper

Directions

Heat oil in a large frying pan. Add eggplant. Fry until golden, then remove and place into a container. In the same frying pan, add onion, garlic, olives, celery, and capers. Cook 5 minutes or until golden. Add more oil if needed, then add tomato sauce, sugar, salt, and eggplant. Toss gently, add vinegar, cover, and cook for 1 minute. Then remove from stove and place in a serving dish.

If you would like to store for 6 months or more, after cooking all the ingredients, get clean glass jars (empty tomato jars are good); fill to the top with caponata and close properly with the metal lid. Place jars in a pan, cover to the top with cold water, bring to a boil, and cook for 25 minutes. Then turn stove off, leave jars in water until it is cold, and then remove jars from water and store in a cool place.

PRAWN SALAD

Servings: 6

Ingredients

500 g fresh cooked, peeled prawns
200 g cooked rice
3 fresh tomatoes, peeled and chopped
1 red pepper, finely chopped
1 stalk celery, finely chopped
2 fresh spring onions, finely chopped
1 tbsp. fresh mint, finely chopped
1 tbsp. fresh parsley, finely chopped
3 tbsp. extra virgin olive oil
2 lemons, cut in 6 wedges
salt and pepper
6 scallop shells

Directions

In large bowl, mix together rice, tomato, pepper, celery, spring onion, mint, olive oil, salt, and pepper. Toss well and fill the scallop shells with this mixed salad. Garnish top with prawn and parsley, and finish with 1 fresh lemon wedge on side.

PEPPERONATA WITH POTATOES

Servings: 6

Ingredients

2 red capsicums, washed, seeded, and cut into strips
2 green capsicums, washed, seeded, and cut into strips
2 yellow capsicums, washed seeded, and cut into strips
3 large potatoes, washed, peeled, and diced
2 large onions, chopped
3 tomatoes, peeled and chopped
olive oil
salt and pepper

Directions

Heat oil in a large frying pan. Add red, green, and yellow capsicum; cook until golden. Then remove and place into a large dish. In the same frying pan, cook potatoes until golden; add more oil if needed. When ready, remove and place with cooked capsicum.

Wash and dry frying pan; return to stove. Heat more oil; add onion and cook until golden. Then add tomato and cook for 5 minutes. Return capsicum and potato to frying pan with the onion and tomato. Add salt and pepper; toss gently, and simmer for 5 minutes. Then remove and serve with your favourite bread.

TOFU PIZZAIOLA

Servings: 6

Ingredients for topping

300 g tofu, cut small
100 g mushrooms, sliced
12 leaves fresh basil
1 large onion, chopped
2 fresh tomatoes, peeled and chopped
1 clove garlic, chopped
1 red capsicum, cut in small pieces
1 yellow capsicum, cut in small pieces
parmesan cheese
extra virgin olive oil
salt and pepper

Ingredients for dough

470 g plain flour
25 g fresh baker's yeast dissolved in 1/2 cup warm water
400ml. warm water
2 tbsp. olive oil
salt

Directions

To make the pizza dough, dissolve fresh yeast in 1/2 cup warm water; stir until dissolved. Put the flour on a flat surface. Make a well in the centre; add the dissolved yeast, salt, 2 tbsp. olive oil, and combine well. Pour in warm water bit by bit and mix well with your hand until it forms sticky dough. Add more flour and knead for a few minutes until the dough is soft, elastic, and smooth. Sprinkle the dough with flour; cover with a tablecloth. Keep warm, and leave to rise for one and a half hours or until doubled in size.

Heat oil in a large frying pan. Add onion, garlic, red and yellow capsicum; cook until golden, then add mushroom, tomato, basil, salt, and pepper. Cook for 10 minutes. Remove from stove and let cool; then add tofu, and toss well.

When dough is ready, roll out into flat circles. Place dough on nonstick oven tray, and add the mixture and tofu. Sprinkle with parmesan cheese and pepper; bake for 25 minutes in 180° C oven until golden and crispy.

VEGETABLE LASAGNE

Servings: 6

Ingredients

200 g instant lasagne
500 g chunky tomato sauce
1 onion, chopped
1 clove garlic, chopped
6 mushrooms, sliced
3 zucchini, sliced
2 red or yellow capsicums, sliced
1/2 cup light mozzarella cheese
2 tbsp. olive oil
salt and pepper

Ingredients for white sauce

500ml. nonfat milk
1/4 cup plain flour
20 g butter

Directions

Heat oil in saucepan. Add garlic and onion; cook until golden, then add vegetables. Cook for 5 minutes. Add tomato, salt, and pepper. Cook uncovered for 10 minutes, then remove from stove.

In saucepan, combine butter, flour, and milk. Bring to a boil and whisk continuously until thickened. Remove from stove.

In a nonstick oven dish, arrange first layer of tomato sauce with veggies, lasagne sheets on top, and white sauce on top of lasagne. Sprinkle with mozzarella cheese. Start next layers by repeating the same process. When ready, bake at 180° C for 45 minutes until top is golden. Then remove from oven, and let stand 15 minutes before serving.

MORTADELLA AND ONION PIZZA WHEELS

Servings: 12

Ingredients

300 g mortadella slices
2 large onions, thinly sliced
4 tbsp. finely chopped parsley
1 cup light mozzarella cheese
olive oil
salt and pepper

Ingredients for dough

470 g plain flour
25 g fresh baker's yeast dissolved in 1/2 cup warm water
400 ml. warm water
2 tbsp. olive oil
salt

Directions

To make the pizza dough, dissolve fresh yeast in 1/2 cup warm water; stir until dissolved. Put the flour on a flat surface. Make a well in the centre; add the dissolved yeast, salt, 2 tbsp. olive oil, and combine well. Pour in warm water bit by bit and mix well with your hand until it forms sticky dough. Add more flour and knead for a few minutes until the dough is soft, elastic, and smooth. Sprinkle the dough with flour; cover with a tablecloth. Keep warm, and leave to rise for one and a half hours or until doubled in size.

When dough is ready, roll out into a few flat rectangular sheets, about 4 or 5 mm thick. Place on top: mortadella, onions, parsley, cheese, salt, and pepper. Roll up dough from the long side, then brush top with oil and cut rolls into 2-cm slices and place cut-side-down on oiled oven tray. Bake in preheated 180° C oven for 20 minutes or until golden.

SPINACH RICOTTA PIZZA WHEEL

Servings: 12

Ingredients

500 g fresh ricotta cheese
200 g fresh spinach, finely chopped
salt and pepper

Ingredients for dough

470 g plain flour
25 g fresh baker's yeast, dissolved in 1/2 cup warm water
400 ml warm water
2 tbsp. olive oil
salt

Directions

To make the pizza dough, dissolve fresh yeast in 1/2 cup warm water; stir until dissolved. Put the flour on a flat surface. Make a well in the centre; add the dissolved yeast, salt, 2 tbsp. olive oil, and combine well. Pour in warm water bit by bit and mix well with your hand until it forms sticky dough. Add more flour and knead for a few minutes until the dough is soft, elastic, and smooth. Sprinkle the dough with flour; cover with a tablecloth. Keep warm, and leave to rise for one and a half hours or until doubled in size.

In a bowl, mix ricotta and spinach, salt, and pepper.

When dough is ready, roll out into flat rectangular sheets about 4 or 5 mm thick. Place ricotta and spinach mixture on top. Roll up dough from long side; then brush top with oil, and cut rolls into 2-cm slices and place cut-side-down on oiled oven tray. Bake in preheated 180° C oven for 20 minutes or until golden.

YUMMY ITALIAN ARANCINE

(Rice balls filled with mozzarella cheese and bolognese sauce)

Ingredients for 60 arancine (the size of tennis balls)

1½ kg rice
350 g breadcrumbs
500 g mozzarella cheese, diced small
2 litres vegetable oil (use only what is needed)
2 beaten eggs
salt

Ingredients for Bolognese sauce

2 bottles chunky tomato sauce, 700 g each
600 g lean minced meat
1/2 cup water
1 onion, finely chopped
1 clove garlic, finely chopped
1 small carrot, finely chopped
1 small celery stalk, finely chopped
300 g peas
2 tbsp. olive oil
1 tbsp. sugar
salt and pepper

Directions

For 60 arancine: boil rice in a large dip saucepan or in two separate pans with plenty of water and salt, for 15 minutes or until soft. When ready, add 1 cup cold water and drain well in a colander; then place rice on flat surface and let cool.

Prepare bolognese sauce by heating 2 tbsp. olive oil in a saucepan. Add onion, garlic, carrot, and celery. Cook until golden, then add minced meat and cook for 5 minutes, stirring well until brown. Add 1 tbsp. wine if you like and let evaporate. Add tomato sauce, sugar, salt and pepper, and 1/2 cup water. Cook for 25 minutes, then remove from stove and let cool.

When rice is cold, add the beaten eggs. Mix well. Place next to rice a container of bolognese sauce, a container of mozzarella cheese, and a container of breadcrumbs. Start rice balls by getting with your left hand half the size of a tennis ball of rice; gently flatten in a cup shape with the help of your right hand, then place in middle 1 square mozzarella cheese and 1 tbsp. bolognese sauce. With your right hand, get another half-size tennis ball of rice. Gently flatten this time with the help of your right hand and place on top your left hand. Gently press and stick together, forming a round tennis ball. Repeat same process with the rest of arancine. Place them separate from each other on a flat surface. Then wash and dry your hands. Start rolling arancine one by one in breadcrumbs, coating balls evenly by holding and pressing very gently in the middle of your two hands. Continue the same process with the rest of the arancine.

Heat vegetable oil in a deep frying pan. Add arancine. When oil is hot, deep fry for 3 minutes or until arancine have a rich golden colour; then remove and drain on paper towels. Serve hot.

FUSILLI PASTA WITH TUNA AND TOMATO

Servings: 6

Ingredients

500 g fusilli pasta
400 g tomatoes, peeled and chopped
185 g tuna in olive oil (Italian style)
1 clove garlic, chopped
1 small onion, finely chopped
4 fillets anchovies
2 tbsp. extra virgin olive oil
parmesan cheese
salt and pepper

Directions

Heat oil in a saucepan. Add garlic, onion, and anchovies. Cook gently until golden. Add tomato, salt, and pepper. Cover and cook for 20 minutes or until sauce is thickened; then add tuna and remove from stove.

Cook pasta by following package directions. Drain well, and serve with sauce and parmesan cheese on top.

FRESH TUNA MARINADE

Servings: 6

Ingredients

6 fresh fillets tuna
300 g fresh tomato, chopped
2 tbsp. fresh basil, chopped
40 g breadcrumbs
12 pitted black and green olives
1 hot chilli, chopped
20 g capers
3 tbsp. extra virgin olive oil
salt and pepper

Directions

Place fillets of tuna in a large nonstick oven dish. Top with breadcrumbs, tomato, basil, green and black olives, capers, hot chilli, olive oil, salt, and pepper. Bake for 35 minutes at 180° C. Serve hot.